From Hair to There

My Personal Journey Through Cancer

Dear Reader

• • •

While this is my story about having a specific cancer, I hope you can all relate it to your own experiences, or those of your loved one. It doesn't matter what it's called, cancer affects our lives in a way like no other, and we are surrounded by people who have either experienced and are cured, or those who are in remission, and those in the middle of battle. We all have a common bond. As you read my story, change the specifics to be your own. Expressing myself in written word is healing for me. I wanted to share it with you.

Warmest wishes to you for a long life filled with happy days. I stand beside you, along with thousands of others. Together we are a vortex of knowledge, courage, solidarity and love.

Know that you are never alone.

-- Linda Trummer

One month after my 60th birthday, I was diagnosed with Blastoid Variant Mantle Cell Lymphoma. MCL is a rare cancer that strikes about 6% of those diagnosed with non-Hodgkin lymphoma. I have the Blastoid variant, which is rarer, with only 2% victimized. I had two days to get a PET Scan and bone marrow biopsy before entering the hospital for my first cycle of aggressive chemotherapy. My treatment plan was 8 cycles, with my odd cycles being R-HyperCVAD, and evens being Rituxan, MTX and ARA-C.

Mantle Cell Lymphoma (CANCER)

listen (MAN-tool sel lim-FOH-muh)

CANCER is an aggressive, fast-growing type of B-cell non-Hodgkin lymphoma (NHL) that usually occurs in adults who are middle-aged or older. It is marked by small- to medium-sized cancer cells that may reside in the lymph nodes, spleen, bone marrow, blood, and/or gastrointestinal system. The blastic variant (BV) form of CANCER is considered a very aggressive subtype of non-Hodgkin lymphoma.

My first stay in the hospital lasted 32 days. I had a reaction to the Rituxan, and cycles 1 and 2 were very difficult on my system. I don't remember too much from those days. I ended my chemotherapy after cycle 6 because my recovery time was too slow. I began a maintenance plan of Rituxan infusions every two months. When I relapse, which will happen as it is part of the beast, my oncologist will first try another chemotherapy combination. Then, we will look for clinical studies

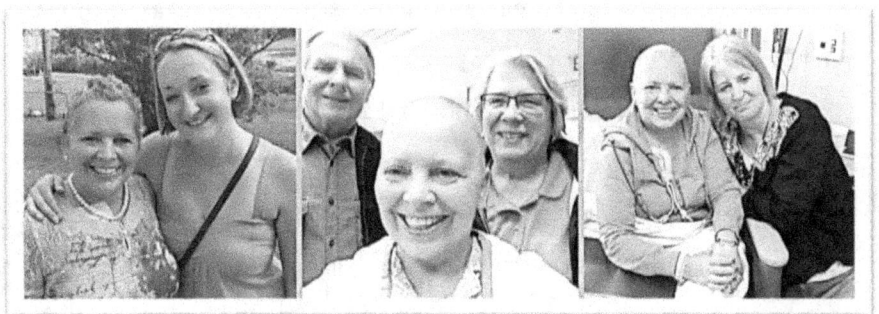

THE IMPORTANCE OF CONNECTING WITH OTHERS

One important thing I've learned is that it doesn't matter what your illness is -- we can all relate. I had this epiphany lying in the hospital, chatting with a visitor who just a year earlier had lung replacement surgery. Until that moment, lost in that conversation, I never thought that he was someone who understood what I was going through. I asked him how he was doing, and he said OK. I told him I thought his color looked good, a sign of health... just to say something, to which he surprised me by replying, "It's my medications." There was that awkward pause while I realized what he said, and then we both laughed out loud, and decided the cosmetics industry should market a make-up for sick people to make them look as badly as they felt.

If you have a serious illness, or are the caretaker of someone who does, never miss the opportunity to connect with like-minded people, and to laugh. Laughter truly is the best medicine.

Your care facility is another place where people connect on an emotional level. I met a couple one day as we were waiting for our turns to get our lab work done. They were about my age, and Shirley had cancer. We chatted for some time, they were a very friendly couple. We hugged as my name was called. Some weeks later, we ran into each other again, and they remembered my name – people passing in time. I didn't think much more of it... until I was readmitted to the hospital for cycle 6 of chemo recently. I was sitting in a family room with another patient, a friend of mine, and his 94-year-old mother and 65-year-old sister. Shirley's husband suddenly entered the room, he had heard my voice. Shirley was back in the hospital with a viral infection. All options were exhausted, and the doctors were talking about moving her to hospice.

I asked if I could stop by to see Shirley, but she was asleep. Later, I wandered down to her room and found her sitting up, visiting with her daughter. They invited me in. I didn't know Shirley's history, but she had lost her hair twice before from chemo, yet it had grown back so beautifully I never would have known her disease had been a part of her life for so long. A disease control doctor had been called in, one who treated me, to help figure out how to get her situation under control. As had happened to me twice before, her immune system had bottomed out and her body had no way to defend itself. The hospice referral was on hold, and there was once again hope. Without her husband present, we could talk about our will to live, and it was obvious that her daughter shared a love with her mother that was giving her the gift of life. I hope Shirley survives. She is a special woman with a loving, supportive family. God bless her.

Then I met Mary, another incredibly lovely woman just a few months' shy of my age. She keeps her head covered and her room sanitized, afraid of the germs that have made her so sick since around Thanksgiving 2015. Her husband is thinking of quitting his job to spend time with his wife, knowing the end may be near. It's these heart-wrenching decisions we all must make, but we find the strength and make them for all the right reasons. Mostly for love.

LOSING YOUR HAIR

I remember waiting for the day my hair would start falling out, and it did. I woke up one morning, and clumps were laying on my pillow. I ran my fingers through my hair, and cried as it fell into my hand, with even more falling out in the shower.

One of the nurses had a good idea – invite my friends to a head shaving party. We snuck a bottle of Hazelnut liqueur into the room and I ordered some

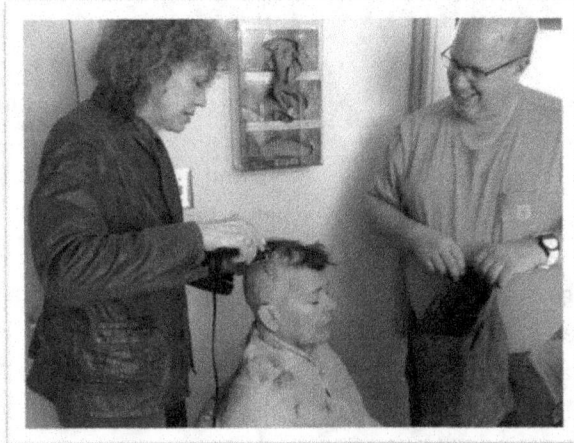

appetizers for us to share. And then I watched in complete horror as several well intended friends shaved my head. It was hideous, but it was a ritual that needed to take place, something I could own. We laughed, and cried, and I stared at my head in horror after everyone had left. It was Rolf who showed up and made this a lifetime memory. He had everything we needed in that bag he brought with him that night and a sense of humor to boot. A couple of days later a stylist came to my hospital room to fix the mess. But, the pictures and the memories are priceless.

At first I kept my head covered, but I never did like hats and such, so I decided being bald was who I was at that moment in time, and I embraced it. Being bald is beautiful -- it means you are alive.

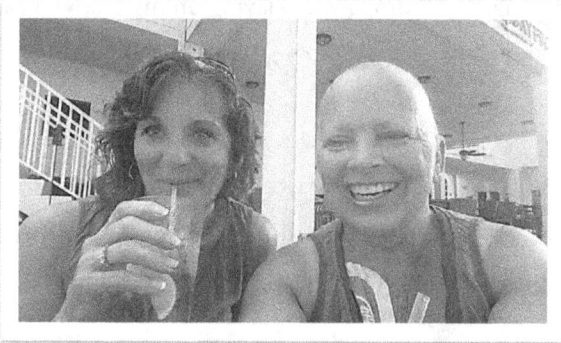

My hubby and I had just gotten married in May 2012 and I was diagnosed in December 2012. Well you know how chemo makes you look. I was bald and pale as pale could be, my eyes sunk in, looking horrible, I told my hubby to leave and he said we got married in sickness and in health, I am staying. Very heartwarming to me. – **Sandy Su, N.C.**

EMBARASSING BODILY FUNCTIONS

Everyone Poops was a children's book written by <u>Tarō Gomi</u> in 1977. Well, not everyone poops. There's nothing like a healthy dose of Dilaudid to clog up one's system. I was on more stool softeners and laxatives than I care to think about. Now, talking about poop might not be the cleanest topic – but it will at least make you chuckle. I was obsessed with pooping, and recently a nurse told me her story. She said as she was prepping me for another treatment that I was particularly stressed about, she decided I deserved some extra Ativan. She suggested that I was already pretty drugged up, but added that a bit more couldn't hurt. A fellow patient and, ironically, a longtime acquaintance, walked into my room. She said I turned to him, and said, "We've got to watch out for these girls, these nurses, because when we're asleep at night, they throw poop at us." She said she waited for me to profess that I was kidding, but I was dead serious.

The first night I woke up with the feeling that I had to poop was the worst. I sat up, climbed off the bed, and to my horror realized my pajama bottoms were filled with, well you know, poop. I managed to get to the bathroom, pulled the call string, and sat and cried while waiting for help. It was a nightmare. Those nurses who came in to help me that first night worked in silence, cleaning me up like I was their baby, and then tucked me back into bed. It happened many times again until I finally realized that I may have needed the pain medications, but I needed my dignity more. I took the high road, and I'll bet the nurses were relieved.

HALLUCINATIONS

In all seriousness, I have had many more imaginary friends in the hospital than reality. And they sure did want to talk to me about something or another!

At first, I would be lying in bed at night, and close my eyes to sleep, when I could see their disembodied faces, familiar yet not, staring at me in the darkness. They were so filled with sadness that I was sure they were long lost cancer victims, and mostly I put straight in my head that I didn't want to listen to nor see them. It was too sad and scary.

It was the man who sat in the recliner who *got* my attention. I could see out of the corner of my right eye his khaki pants and work boots. That was all. He would sit in that chair and cross his legs. When I looked, thinking my son was visiting, there was nothing but an empty chair.

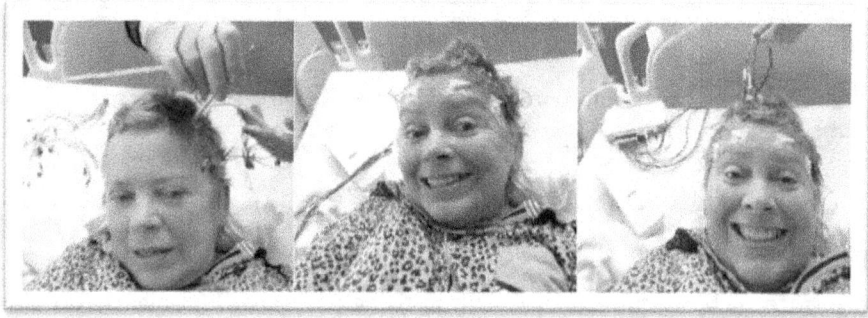

Then he moved to the wall directly in front of my bed. Still, I could only see his khaki pants and work boots, but he started talking to me. I mostly ignored him and the others who were shy about showing themselves, but sometimes you just need to answer!

During one of my son's visits, I spotted a large black creature on the ceiling, so I asked what it was. My son couldn't see it, so I got up to point to it. It was huge and just hovering -- but it wasn't real.

I later learned that I had hypoactive delirium, which caused hallucinations and a variety of other symptoms. The condition flared on a hospital stay for an infection around Mother's Day. My short-term memory was shot, and my hallucinations turned grander and rather frightening. At one point, I imagined a hospital technician had approached me to remove my Hickman. I was surprised and told her, no, I wasn't done with it.

The conversation that followed made no sense, and I finally told her she needed to speak with my nurse. I also told my nurse, who went to look for this mysterious person. She returned to tell me the woman had made a mistake and would return to apologize to me. It wasn't until nearly a month later when I was reporting this story to another nurse that it was suggested I had imagined the entire incident. I was shocked, but it was likely that it was a mind trick during my delirium.

TRAVELING WITH CANCER

On a recent trip to Florida, my friends took me out to dinner during the trip, and we happened into a local bar/restaurant. It was very small with a giant pool table and bar area. Four women stood by the bar and watched as we were seated at a high-top table, I assumed the women were staring at the good looking young man who accompanied us, so imagine my surprise when the first woman approached me.

When you often go out hairless, you forget, it's who we are when undergoing chemo. Some of us embrace it, as I do. So, we forget that we kind of stand out in a crowd. Anyway, this young woman came up to me and hugged me, with no warning, and thanked me and whispered words of encouragement, and all I could do was hug her back and wait for what might come next. I could feel her emotion, and she was quite shaken as she stepped away long enough for woman number 2 to do the same.

I must have happened upon a very personal moment that these women were sharing, and cancer was our common denominator. Woman number 3 was next, hugs and thoughtful words, and woman number 4 friends while telling me that I was going to beat this, and giving me a thumbs-up. I noticed woman number 1 was visibly shaken by this encounter, and I knew that it was her moment I had become a part of, and her friends were there for moral support. To become a part of someone else's story, especially something as incredibly personal and emotional as cancer, is a truly a privilege. To have four strangers approach me in such a way honestly took my breath away. I was honored, and will remember this for a long time to come. I don't know how they will remember the experience, but it brings tears to my eyes for many reasons and on many levels. It wasn't the first time, and I'm sure it won't be the last.

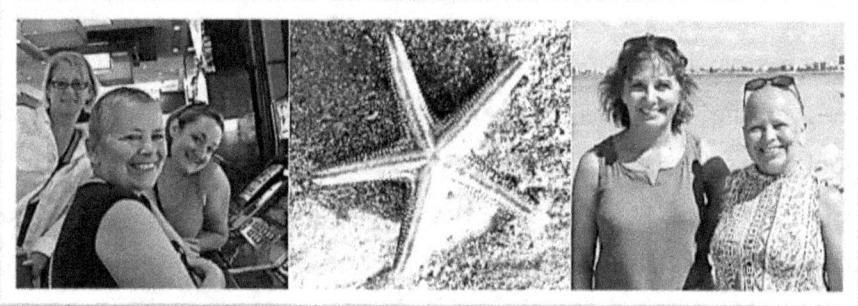

As for those high-top tables, up until that outing I had avoided them, certain they were going to cause me problems... and they did. After sitting at one for a couple of hours, my legs stopped working properly and I couldn't get off that chair for the life of me. My friends had to literally lift me off the chair and help me regain my balance so we could leave.

While in Orlando, we took two day trips to the beach. Wear something on your head to the beach. The first time I wore a lazy looking black hat. I had to hold that darn thing on the whole afternoon. The second trip I wore a wig and a hat. The hat flew off, but that faithful wig stuck to my head, all afternoon. The sweat it caused likely helped it stay stuck. But WOW, the pictures look great. No worries about whether I had cancer, nor any doubt that something was medically wrong with me. My Hickman line, or catheter dressing shows very visibly from my upper chest. The Florida sunshine felt good, and if a cancer patient is well enough to travel, do it, with or without hair.

To wear a wig or not – I sure do wish I hadn't worn it on the return flight. It's uncomfortable and I wanted to whip it off my head several times. There's no need for explanation to anyone when one goes hairless. It's cancer. It doesn't matter how anyone else feels, I have cancer. Smile and be nice, ignore me, I don't care. Just move out of my way, especially when I have pain and don't feel well.

As I headed home to Minneapolis, I pre-boarded the plane. A mother and teenaged daughter sat next to me. Not once did I say a word to them in conversation. By the time we arrived home, I found myself so exhausted that my legs weren't working well, a neurological problem I often experience now. Suddenly I heard a voice come from my right side, "Would you like an arm to hold on to?" It was the woman who had been sitting next to me for the past 3 hours. I started to cry, I was so overwhelmed by the kind gesture. I took her arm and thanked her, as she handed my heavy backpack to her daughter. They were both so gracious and kind. We walked to the baggage carousel together, where they had me sit while they waited for my plaid suitcase to come tumbling down. Once they were sure my son was on his way, they bid me good night and were gone. Yet, another miracle.

"You gain strength, courage, and confidence by every experience in which you really stop to look fear in the face. You must do the thing which you think you cannot do."

- Eleanor Roosevelt.

MANY PEOPLE ARE AFFECTED BY CANCER

Such kindness finds me wherever I go. Cancer affects many people, and creates kindred spirits across the globe. I have been touched by strangers in miraculous ways. The first stranger experience was in a small gift shop. A woman about my age walked up to me, hugged me, and blessed me with luck for a healthy recovery. Her daughter was a breast cancer survivor. I learned that I would continue to unwittingly walk into other people's personal moments. If you open your heart, you are a receptor for such opportunities.

*My husband was diagnosed with cancer over 12 years ago, and ever since, I keep a daily list of precious memories I scroll through & visualize whenever the clouds of depression or waves of panic and fear start to envelop me. A few days ago, we were told he was tp53 deleted and the battle would be that much harder. Six years ago, he beat the odds and survived a Richter's Transformation of his CLL (DLBCL). Miracles can happen. I've come to see each day as a miracle. Another opportunity to experience joy, but if it's a day filled with fear or panic or depression, I force myself to visualize the precious memories we've been making and remind myself how blessed we were to have that moment in time. It's not always easy...and I admit I'm not always successful but I choose to not allow myself to dwell in my own personal darkness too long. Yesterday, we took our 5-year-old grandson to his first professional baseball game. It was a perfect day in every way and this moment will be added to my list to comfort us on dark days. Although I do not know you personally, Linda, your open & honest words have been an inspiration to me. I truly hope you write that book. The world needs it. (((Hugs))) – **Stella***

Everyone has his or her own personal story; none of us are on the exact same journey. But there is a common thread woven throughout that brings us to a common place, and we're only alone if we want to be.

When I was in remission from Nov. 2013 to Feb. 2016, I used to joke (but half-seriously) with my wife, "I never had cancer; it was just some crazy misdiagnosis or bad dream I had." Even when I was first diagnosed and home from hospital the first time (I spent a month in hospital when first diagnosed) and in recovery mode after a couple of weeks, I used to lie in bed and think I was just fine, nothing had changed, no therapy ahead. I think we want to get back to the place we were before diagnosis, when we didn't have the looming angel of death tethered to us like a kite, following along above and behind, even though we all (healthy or not) do. But, I guess, like several have commented, each of us ha to find those people, those moments, those places, things, experiences and what-have-you that help us to get through and find joy, whether we're healthy or not. I know today I'm going to climb up a ladder and clean out the gutters—that will make my wife happy. **Mark, Michigan**

FINDING KNOWLEDGE

In the beginning, I was so eager to learn about my illness, to find others who shared my experiences. I went to the American Cancer Society and the Leukemia and Lymphoma Society sites. One brilliant day, I typed my disease into the search line of Facebook and instantly found the place I wanted to be. At first it was like a head rush, hearing from nearly 1,200 people what it was like to have MCL. Mostly, they talked about Stem Cell Transplants. It was like the latest brand of jeans, or a trendy new restaurant that everyone needed to go to. Finally, once I was to the point of either staying in the group or leaving, I posed the question: "Is there anyone in here who hasn't had Stem Cell Transplant (SCT)?" At first my question was met with dead silence, like it was taboo to say they had not. And then slowly people started speaking up, telling their stories of why they had not, and they became bolder as more and more people stepped forward. The room was finally in sync.

There is great comfort to being in a support group, where people share a commonality. Of course, not all of us will have the same treatment, side effects, or future, but we can still relate.

And when we lose a warrior to cancer, we mourn together, like family. When we have success, we celebrate. I've made many new friends this way, people who even on my worse days know what I'm experiencing. To have such support is priceless.

HOW THE HECK DOES ONE WRITE A BOOK?!

I have not been sleeping well, most of my posts in the on-line support room were pre-dawn, and someone suggested including them in this book. Each one of the following writings is a stage I went through during my treatment. I hope they resonate with you.

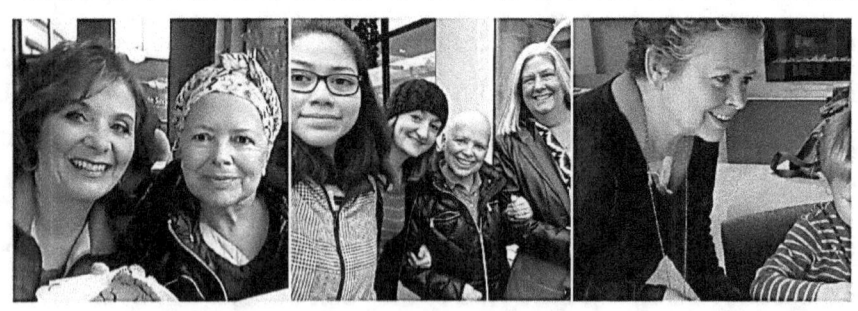

My Journal of Thoughts

♥   Chemotherapy, or "chemical treatment," has been around since the days of the ancient Greeks. However, chemotherapy for the treatment of cancer began in the 1940s with the use of nitrogen mustard. I guess I didn't know the history. But I know the present. As I lie in bed with this chemical treatment flowing through my veins, I think of how trusting we are that this even works. It kills everything in sight, and I can feel the effects of it in my achy leg bones this morning. I anticipated this would happen - even brought my walker, just in case. I am now 8 hours away from being done with this cycle. I am scheduled to go home tomorrow morning - not sure I can wait until then. I'm going to try to be set free this afternoon. I want to go home. I miss home.

♥   Well, friends, I'm back in the hospital, just 3 days after my 5th cycle of chemo. My best friend brought me in at 4:40 am Tuesday. I woke up about 4 am and felt icky. Took my temperature and it was 103. (They always tell us to head to the Emergency Room with a temp of 100.3 or higher.) Same thing happened after cycle 4. To make matters worse, the MRI from yesterday shows something on my brain that must be dealt with, sooner than later. I'm sorry to report that my legs aren't working right, so I can't dance. Therefore -- I'm counting on each of you to turn on your favorite dance song - and dance like there's no tomorrow.

♥   I started my first 24-hour cycle of Doxorubicin and it hit me hard. My mood dropped in a flash, and it zapped the energy out of me. I will have two more of such bags, and be done by Thursday afternoon - possibly go home then or Friday. I've been fortunate, though, with high energy and good spirits up until now - and even feeling better this morning. A fellow was watching me flutter about yesterday, and finally came into my room to say he was intrigued by me. He was a chaplain, and he asked if he could sit and talk. He eventually asked me a deeply personal and spiritual question: "Who are you? Who are you really?" I told him I wasn't far enough along in my thought process to know the answer. He then shared a quote, and said, this is who you are: "You aren't a human being having a spiritual experience; you are a spiritual being having a human experience." It made me cry, but they were good tears.

♥   Life was so much easier pre-cancer. Right? It seems so long ago, and I'm wondering if it was easier, or if it's just a false memory. I think I was still tired and anxious and crabby, but for different reasons. Mostly, I worked long hours and didn't spend a whole lot of time enjoying life. Now it's like everything is right next to the surface, and whether it's a good feeling or pain, it's raw emotion that can remind you how glad you are to be alive, or how close you might be to death. The turn of every corner teaches you something new, introduces you to someone you never would have known, or brings into your life an unexpected miracle. Maybe we're more alive now than ever before. Maybe this is the biggest blessing of all, our most difficult challenge, the fight for our life... I wonder.

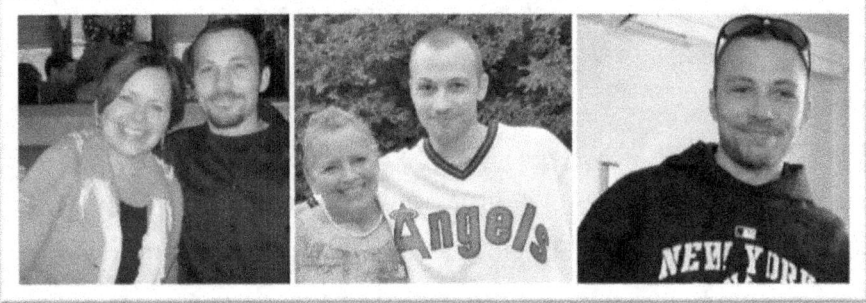

♥   My son is getting much better at making a great cup of coffee. Either that or my taste buds are getting less discerning. I choose to believe the coffee is better. My son has done so much for me over the past 8 months. I'm sure those of you with caregivers can agree that having someone who loves you help you through this is a gift. My sister is another person who continues to be a supportive influence in my life with cancer. She runs her own business, has her own family plus grandchildren, yet I know she thinks of me every day, and sees me when she can. We learned to skype together - which was rather hilarious. But every night while I was in the hospital those first 32 days, we had virtual chats. And then there's my best friend -- I am so blessed to have such caring people in my life. It lightens the load; don't you think? Cheers to those of you who are caregivers and thank you for loving us, even on our bad days. This wouldn't be a journey without you - it would be a prison sentence. Love & Hugs

♥   I'll miss the sunshine, but can't you just hear the grass growing on a day like today (Spring 2016)? I had a PET Scan yesterday, and my doctor's nurse called late afternoon to let me know everything is still clear. It's been that way since my second cycle of chemo. I hope my platelets are up by tomorrow so I can begin cycle six of 8. Today is going to be a Rock & Rollin' kind of day -- getting the music going so I can wake it up and shake it up a bit. Cheers, my friends!

♥   My platelets dropped, from 84 - 71, from Monday to today, but my oncologist spoke with her colleagues and they decided if I was willing to take the risk of bleeding, they would decrease my treatment and add a few precautions - so I was admitted to the hospital for cycle 6 today. If things don't go well, this will be my last before beginning maintenance.

♥   Of course, the medical staff would be happy if I could complete 8 cycles of chemo, but we'll see how things go. I'm feeling optimistic. To me it's better to take a physical risk than the emotional one caused by all these delays. And so, we will begin with Rituxan today. My platelets have prevented me from a regular schedule, and it is time to just take a risk and hope for the best. I'd lie if I said I wasn't a wee bit worried, but I know my body well. If anything is amiss, I'll be reporting it. So.... let the treatment begin.

♥   My friends, I had to tell you some good news today. My blood test results are back - I'm an early riser and get early results. By today, we expected my counts would drop - but they didn't! They ALL went up, even my platelets are at 79. My nurse thinks it's the fluids infusion that are helping. I am half way through a 22-hour bag of Meth TX. I know it's a small victory, but I'm hoping for the best. Remember, I came in with low platelets, and the doctor was concerned but we decided to give it a try. The only two side effects I'm experiencing are bladder control and headaches. Yes, I'm wearing big girl diapers - not ashamed to admit it. Makes for a good chapter in my book.

♥   My 3rd bag of chemo at 1:30 am, and now I'm wide awake. I think I failed the pre-test, where I must walk toe to toe and such. They woke me from a drug induced sleep, and I can't remember half of what I did - but know they had to call the on-call doctor to see if I could begin the chemo. Stupid rules. The good news of the day is that my Methotrexate levels are nearly normal, which means I should be able to go home tomorrow. The big conversation will be if I will be able to convince my doctor to continue my final two chemo cycles, which I think will be a long-term benefit to me, rather than quitting and starting maintenance. We shall see how that debate goes.

♥   It's with bitter sweetness that I am ending my chemotherapy with cycle 6, which I'm just completing, rather than finishing my original prescribed 8 cycles. My counts just aren't recovering fast enough in between cycles, and doctor and her colleagues are recommending I stop at 6 and begin my maintenance plan of Rituxan every two months, with labs 3 x a week. I have grown so fond of the medical staff I've worked with at the hospital, and will miss them a lot. But, I'm becoming a member of the hospital's Patient Family Partnership Council to help improve patient care, and I'm also hoping to help start an art program to bring bored patients together to work on projects that will be therapeutic in many ways - art is a great way to engage people in meaningful conversation that can be so healing. Just thinking of my own hours being tethered to 24 hour bags of chemo with nothing productive to do makes me think art would be a great way to engage people during these long hours of hospital imprisonment. Anyway, I came into this final cycle with low platelets, with risks involved - but I made it through. Need to get my Meth TX levels down just a wee bit more to wrap things up, and I'll head home late this afternoon. I've got a good life to come - I know it. Short or long, it will be the best. Still have a lot of dancing to do!

♥ Good morning, everyone. I didn't sleep well last night, but I sure had no hardship waking up. I wanted to thank you all for your love and support over these past few days. I couldn't make it far without you - you all give so much during such a challenging time. I'm heading in this morning for lab work, but I can tell by that weakness in my legs that my counts are already beginning to drop. I won't see my oncologist for a few more weeks to determine what my plan of action will be. But the good news is my bucket list has a few things in it, some still secret because they affect my future quite substantially, but a couple that are for fun. I'm making plans to head to Ft. Myers Beach with my sister - her first trip there. We'll leave June 1 for 9 days on the beach.

♥ Dawn came with no singing birds today, causing my heart to feel empty and sad. I sat and listened more intently, wondering ... What could be the trouble on such a crisp early morning? Maybe a storm, perhaps too cold? I rubbed my sleepy eyes and sat up straight in bed and for a moment held my breath. Surely there was something wrong that the birds overslept. I silenced my mind, willing with all my might the day to come alive, and then I heard. A dog bark. A car passing. And then the most beautiful sound of all -- a bird chirping outside my window. Sometimes we are so set to the sounds happening – anticipating the mundane or fullness of each day that it's internally a challenge to hear and see the beauty of nature, of the grander design of life. And it's not right or wrong. Hearing and feeling what's important in each moment is what makes life so precious. My heart can ache

20

or it can sing, like that morning bird, and that will be who I am. Today it will sing.

♥   What exactly is the meaning of life? I never thought much about it before, but I woke up this morning thinking, really, what the heck is it? Or are we just part of a microcosm of relatively intelligent life that just happened to be? An illusion or reality? Perhaps it will remain a mystery, or maybe we know once we reach our next destination, when we're all called into a giant conference room and given the secrets to the complicated life we've been living, and the reasons why. I'm not a religious person, but I do believe in God. I also believe that death is not the end, that God has a plan for His children. With such a belief, - how can we be afraid?

♥   Good morning from my hospital bed. My White Blood Count (WBC) dropped to 0.1 and platelets were 6, now climbed to 14 after 2 transfusions. My highest fever has been 103, it's climbing again this morning. My nurse reminded me I need to stay alive until Valentine's Day 2017 because we're going out on the town - cool chick style. Just to be clear, I certainly hope to be alive beyond Feb 2017, but it does give me something to add to my bucket list, which is designed to keep me forward moving. In between extreme teeth-chattering shivers, I'm working on plans for my future, and there's a lot to do when one is 60 - not quite retirement age, and needing to plan for the financial future. I didn't think about all of that when I was younger, and am lucky to have a great financial advisor who is also a friend - he has my best interests at heart.

♥   Finally, the rain has stopped. I hope I didn't just jinx it -- but I am tired of rainy days. I need some sunshine! There is something about the healing qualities of the sun, sitting outdoors and feeling the warmth soaking into your skin. Unlike chemo... by quite a bit, don't you think? I've been feeling the poison traveling through my veins, and have spent much of the past 3 days since I've been home from the hospital in bed -- tired and sick. Maybe I've been thinking this all wrong. Instead of being afraid of stopping my chemotherapy a couple cycles early, I should be rejoicing that I have this chance to cleanse my body, to start anew. On insane days, I wonder if I have cancer at all, and I think maybe once the chemo has finished its final flow through my veins, it will wash with it the cancer, that I'll wake up one morning cancer free. With a full head of hair, to boot! And thirty years younger, and 30 pounds thinner... famed author of the world's greatest book on cancer, entitled -- oh, let's just call it, From Hair to There. And from my mansion in the hills of somewhere, we'll be having a party, and we'll all be cancer free and live happily ever after. See what a sunny day can do, or is it my hypo delirium sneaking back? Oh, who cares?! Happily, EVER after!!

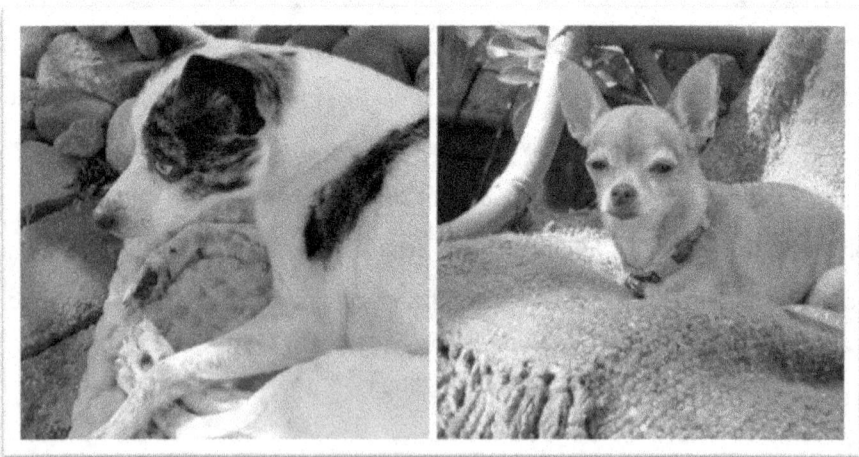

♥ I'm waking next to my old dog who is snoring like an old man. Isn't it amazing how much pleasure our pets can give us? I've got a Chihuahua who sleeps to the left of me, and a Jack Russell sleeping to my right -- and an occasional cat or two that gets a what-for-all when she tries to climb up next to the warmth of my bedding. The sun is shining this morning - perhaps the rain is postponed for a bit, I hope. I'm heading in soon to get my labs done, and to keep my coveted appointment with my psychoanalyst. I don't feel the best today, but I sure am happy that I have so many things to look forward to doing in the months to come.

♥ I want to go to the nursery tomorrow and dig in the soil ... get my fingernails dirty as I fill my planters with fresh new plants that will beautify my backyard. And then I want to throw all my medications away, cleansing my veins from all this poison and hope for wellness. But first I'll have my Hickman removed and never ever have blood drawn again. I want to swim underwater and take a shower without having to worry about getting things wet. And I want to plug in my blow dryer and curling iron and get out all my hair products. I don't want to clean the cat litter pans, but I would if it made my cancer go away. It's exhausting, don't you think, this illness that will likely kill us, especially those of us with Blastoid Variant? I'm awake when I should be asleep, and asleep when I shouldn't be. I can't remember my beautiful, colorful dreams anymore, and children stare at me in the grocery store because I have no hair. My cats have either gained or lost weight, and my dogs cower every time I pull out my suitcase. One pisses on the rug, and the other just looks mournful and sleeps close to me at night so he can be sure to know if my breathing changes. I don't want my friends to cry, or my

23

relatives to feel the need to call me, and I don't want to sit around the house because I don't feel well. I want to go for long walks and go dancing and flirt - and be flirted with. I don't want cancer, but since I do, I want to find a cure. How about you?

♥ Good Morning, friends! After a weird but restful sleep with night sweats and such, I'm again awake at 4 am - ready to face another day. Lovely to hear the birds singing outside my window. Have you noticed - even on days with no appointments, there are phone calls to make, paperwork to complete regarding disability, etc.? It seems endless, and complex. I'm sure glad my bout with hypo delirium is over so I can think clearly again. I found a wonderful quote to share.

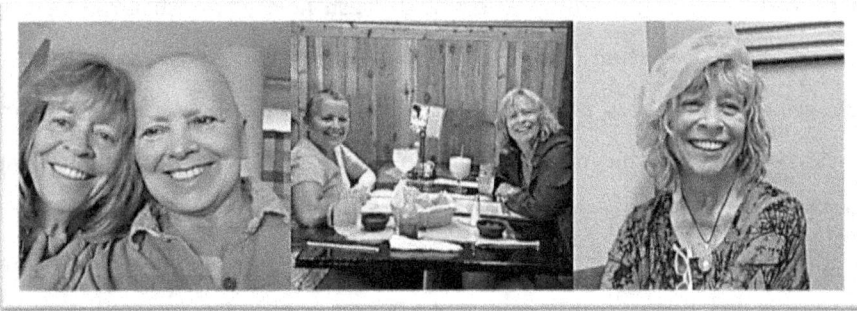

♥ My best friend and I have started having end-of-life conversations, with great respect for our relationship that is close to 30 years young. Never ever when we first met did we think we'd be having these talks, much less how important they would be. But, regardless of how much time I have left, I don't want to miss a single moment or a single word. Of course, I can be positive and hope to live forever. But if I'm gone in the blink of an eye, nothing should be left unsaid nor a special moment uncaptured. I think I'm becoming a more patient person, savoring each minute of life, for better or worse;

having delicious conversations, noticing every bird that sings, and the loving way my dogs and cats look at me, especially when I'm eating a particularly good piece of meat. See -- never miss a chance to throw in a pun or a bit of humor or even sarcasm. My life is filling up with everything I ever imagined, and I'm in love with living it. When it's done, it's done -- but for now, I'm not going to miss one word, one smile, or one single hug, or the love of a friend. Win-Win for me!

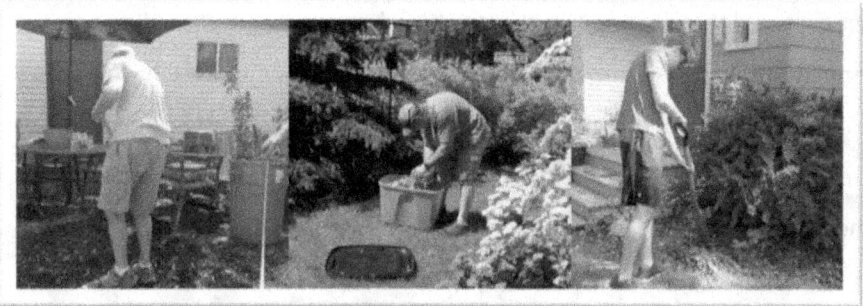

♥   My wish for filled flower pots, a weeded yard, and a planted garden finally came true today. 7 friends arrived this morning to do yardwork and I grilled brats to feed them. I am so amazed with how hard they worked and how much was accomplished in just a couple hours. I love my friends.

♥   I was reminded by what someone said, that we do now live life in limbo. I don't think that's a negative thought, but rather the reality of what cancer has brought to our lives. There is a fine balance between life and death, regardless, and we must think of one to accept the other. When will we die? How will it feel? Both natural questions when struck by a cancer with deadly intentions, questions that we will likely revisit more than once. I was diagnosed with Blastoid Variant MCL 8 months ago, and I still wonder... but in between, life goes on and we must travel with it. This is our journey, and there is no right or wrong way to live with cancer. It's easy to say, keep a positive attitude, or live one day at a time. And hopefully most days we can stay on that track, but some -- and it will vary for us each -- we will think about dying, and it's a part of the grieving process that ultimately keeps us healthy. I'd like to think I have 3, 5, 10 or 12 years to go -- as some of you have shared. But I want them to be good years, not years filled with sickness or sorrow. As some of you know, I have my bucket list, and it's filling up. Most days, it's that list and figuring out how best to accomplish all the things I want to during this lifetime. But in between, I might -- no, I will have a down moment where I wonder about dying, and I hope on those days, during those moments, I will be near someone who will let me be in my private thoughts, someone who might hug me or allow me to engage in an open conversation about it. Knowing my friends, I'm certain that will be the case -- and once it's out of my system, my otherwise good day will continue until next time. Limbo. A terrible place to be, unless you can accept it as part of our journey.

♥ Good morning, friends. Well, I had a follow up visit with the oncology psychiatrist -- a subject that's a bit uncomfortable for me to talk about. But it's a reminder to us all that we must take care of our mental and emotional well-being as well as our physical throughout our journey with cancer. When I was hospitalized this last time with fevers and pneumonia, I knew something was wrong, and I asked to speak with this doctor. I was diagnosed with hypo delirium, brought on by the fevers. For me, it was a short-term memory loss -- felt like, if you will, my mind was a slide show, and there were slides missing that made things distorted - and kind of frightening. Yesterday, as I visited with the doctor, I began to cry - for no reason - and then I told him I was still forgetful, having night sweats, and dreaming of trying to organize cancer-related appointments, treatments and such. He then understood that my problems were cognitive, that I still had low-grade delirium, but that I needed to find clarity and order in my life. He prescribed a baby dose of Ritalin, which he hopes will help. I'm sharing this with you all because I want to express the importance of recognizing that this isn't just a physical journey, but one of our whole being - and don't be afraid to ask for help when you need it.

♥   Each morning when I awaken my vision is blurred for about 2 hours. I literally close one eye to be able to see clearly. Mostly I just type away with the blurriness, hoping something spectacular is written that I never would have come up with otherwise. I was just thinking what a glorious morning it is. I'm feeling good, my head is on straight, and I do believe I will enjoy the day. I hope upon hope that everyone in this room will join me. Let's enjoy the beauty that spring has brought us -- it's a gift to enjoy. And listen to those birds sing -- filling the air with a symphony, for free. My peonies are blooming, as are a million other things in my yard. We're alive. Life is good. A great day to dance.

"It's only when we truly know and understand that we have a limited time on earth - and that we have no way of knowing when our time is up - that we will begin to live each day to the fullest, as if it was the only one we had."

Elisabeth Kübler-Ross Hoyt

♥ For sure, don't wake up in the middle of the night for a drink of water and keep the water in bed with you... unless you like lying in ice water. How this happens? Sleeping medication or just plain stupidity... who knows.

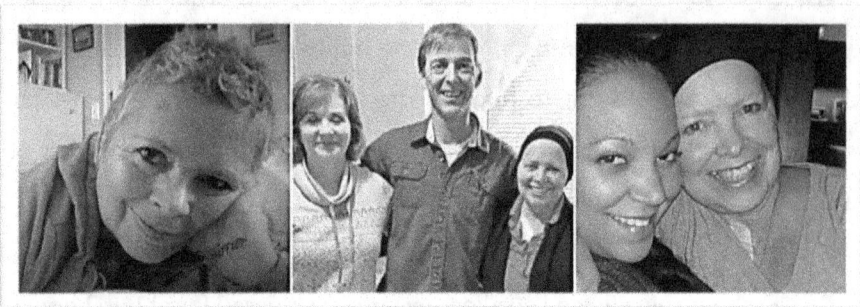

It is a good excuse to change your bed linens, which I've been meaning to do anyway. Don't you wish you could take the nursing assistant home with you to tend to such matters? For all the times, I said, no, you don't need to change the sheets today. I should have asked for a rain check. Will they even make house calls -- likely not? Honestly, by the time I'm done doing it myself now that I'm home, I need a nap, I'm so winded.

♥ Remember when we were kids and we had a quarter to go to the candy store? I remember walking back and forth in front of that case, looking at all the candy and calculating just how much I could buy for 25 cents. When I finally made my choice, I paid my money and left with my brown paper bag filled with sugary treasures. I would find a tree, sit and lean against it and enjoy my treats. I can remember lying on my back and watching the clouds roll by, finding elephants and bears and all kinds of figures floating through the sky. It's funny how these memories came to me this morning as I was walking on the beach and suddenly found myself struggling to breath. I think it was the barometric pressure -- the weight in the air following the storm. I just couldn't catch my breath, and my legs felt like lead -- and I was all alone.

I looked at the ocean slapping water up against my feet, which I could only slide to keep myself going, and I thought how magnificent and powerful the waves were, and how as a child I played in the water for hours on end. Crap -- I thought -- was I going to die walking on the beach? Where were all these long-ago memories coming from? Is this what it's like before life ends. I couldn't do that to my sister... I could no longer pick up my feet, so I slid them along the wet morning sand, thinking of penny candy and cloud dragons, and playing in the water until I made it back to our building... and I made it to the elevator... and I made it. My breathing is once again normal, and the sun is shining. Another day to cherish. Love to you all.

♥   Are there any survivors of cancer was the question, and the answer from those of us who have cancer is a resounding YES! We are alive and we are survivors, and we plan to keep surviving if possible. I'm a survivor with Blastoid variant, which creates more of a challenge, and I'm also a survivor who will not be having SCT, either auto or allo. I have a bucket list that is getting so full that I'm going to have to live for a very long time to complete it, and I can't imagine not finishing each one. Are there any survivors - and, yes, I know what the question meant? I am 60 years old, nearly 61, come August 29. My doctor predicts 18 - 24 months for me, and I call that BS because it's not enough time. So... I'll prove her wrong, and if I don't, I honestly believe there is an afterlife that will be so amazingly beautiful, and we can live happily ever after, eternally.

♥   Do you ever for just a moment or two forget that you have cancer? And does that moment feel like nothing ever changed -- that it's just another Friday night and another ordinary day? I do, from time to time - lying on my bed catching up on what my FB friends are up to, going out to dinner with friends, or doing nothing just like every other ordinary person I know. Sometimes I feel just a bit guilty because I've forgotten that I'm not the only one who is trying so very damn hard to live in the moment. My friend Michael lost his mother this week - not to cancer, but to age. One of my friends who volunteered to help with yardwork a few weeks ago had a lung transplant last year, and I almost forgot to make sure he was okay as he dug in the soil, planting things. I guess we sometimes forget that the world doesn't revolve around us and our illness -- that there are still 7.4 billion people on planet earth and each in his or her own way is struggling through a life experience, possibly not but seemingly so as challenging as ours. So far today there were 151,480 deaths. Each year 12.7 million people discover they have cancer and 7.6 million people die from the disease. And on June 10, 2016, every one of us is alive. Just another Friday night... I am thankful.

♥   I started today what is referred to as cancer rehab - exercise, strengthening, etc. I'll be going twice a week. I look forward to good results. Also, the art program I've started with cancer patients at my hospital continues to go well. It's amazing how powerful the conversations are over a simple art project. Today I met a woman whose mother went in with colon cancer, and it's spread so much that she's expected to die. This woman has been trying to manage her mother's care and deal with 10 out of country siblings, and having someone to talk with lightened her load. She's also been getting different advice from different specialists, and had never heard of Palliative Care, which we gave her information about. I also spent some time with a four-year-old and her father. Grandma didn't have cancer, but rather Hep C from her alcoholism. Lots of anger involved here, but a bit of coloring brought on some smiles. Next Thursday I start my maintenance regime of

Rituxan every other month. Looking forward to giving it a try. Feeling optimistic.

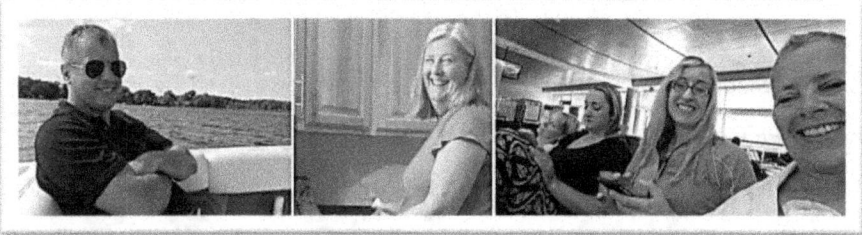

♥   In many ways, it's been a blessing to me, one that has forced me to recognize and appreciate friends and family, and each single day of life. I've also had time to realize I'm a lot stronger than I thought, and that I'm kind of proud of the woman I've grown into through life experiences these past 60 years. If I die tomorrow, I have left nothing undone. I'm not going to lie - this diagnosis was given to me as a death sentence. I didn't need to Google life expectancy -- my oncologist told me. Maybe I'm foolish - but I feel like I'm going to live forever. Since my last chemo cycle, I've gotten stronger, feeling better about whatever lies before me. Everyone should live as though tomorrow was our last day – make us think about what matters most. I would live that day as I'm living today. Now, that is a blessing.

♥   I'm waking up too early from crazy dreams and night sweats, and I feel like I've been hit by a semi-truck, to boot. Just how did that vice grip manage its way inside my chest, and all the while the start to a Jim Reeves song keeps playing over and over in my head -- "Welcome to my world... won't you come on in..." I'm thinking it's the new medication that is supposed to not only help me sleep better, but control my anxiety. Must be "opposite day" somewhere. Oh, well, we'll just try to make the best of this -- nothing a few games of Facebook Gin Rummy won't cure.

♥ Sleepless in Minnesota. My liver enzymes are rising dramatically. I have a PET scan at 6:45 am, to rule out - or not - that it's related to cancer. I need to get in to see my GI doctor so she can do her tests. I was diagnosed early on in this whole process with Hepatitis C, and there's a possibility that the chemo triggered it. My new health insurance year starts today, which means new deductibles. I'm a little bit stressed. But, it's not as though I haven't been through these little side trips before. Just another day with cancer. The part that's a bit unnerving is that I can't continue with anymore treatment for the cancer until my liver problem is stabilized.

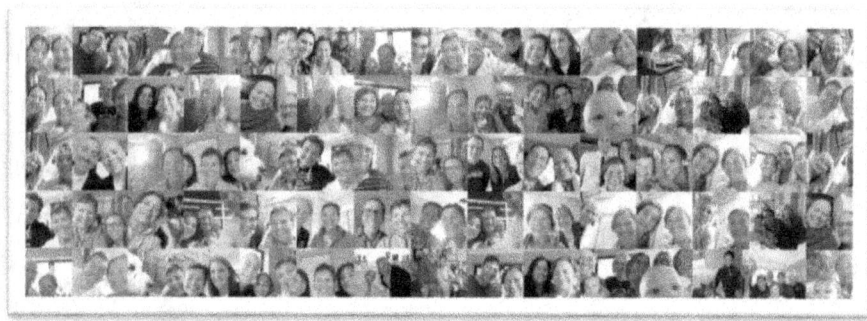

♥ My friend with, same as me, Blastoid variant MCL has relapsed for the second time in a few short months. Most recently it's been only a month from chemo. He's trying to do what many think is the right thing to do, have SCT. I understand there are differing levels of success with SCT, and many of you swear it's the only way to go. He will now undergo yet 1 to 2 more rounds of HyperCVAD in hopes of remission and a third try at SCT. After a while, what is the cost to our bodies? While there is promising, new research posted in here each day, ultimately some of us will die from this disease. I'm not suggesting we give up hope, but we must make mindful and practical decisions about what is reasonable for us as individuals. Collectively, we can have conversations and support one another, which is the beauty of this room. There are varied opinions and much wisdom. Set your respective goals. If long life is your goal, try it all until something works. But ask the questions of your oncologist to make sure all angles are being considered. Quality of life is important, too. I write this with love and respect.

♥   I know I'm taking a risk by writing today - but some days aren't about having positive thoughts and being hopeful. That day is today for me. I've had much time to think about my life, and I don't like how I'm living right now. I miss my healthy years, feel like I lost a piece of my identity. I realize that to many of you, I'm still a new kid on the block. I had my first biopsy in early August of 2015. I'm working hard to rebuild who I am. But so much has happened these past 11 months that some days I can't wrap my head around it. I must say it was easier for me when first diagnosed - followed by a whirlwind of treatment and delirium and fear. Why? Because I was in the hospital and taken care of and didn't have much energy to think, just follow directions. I'm in physical therapy to strengthen my body, meeting a counselor to talk about feelings, and volunteering at the hospital to keep busy and feel I have something to give back. Still, something is missing for me - and I don't have a better way to describe it. I'll most likely feel better tomorrow - maybe not. But sometimes don't you just feel like saying it like it is, even if it's just for today?

♥   I am usually good about asking for a ride when I'm feeling over fatigued. Well, this morning I underestimated how poorly I was feeling, and jumped in my car for an appointment with the endocrinologist. I didn't realize how badly things were going until on the way home -- when I passed out and slammed into the rear of another car. Fortunately, neither of us were injured and he was very kind. But there was a guy in a pickup who had been following me, and told me I had been driving up on the curb, barely missing trees, etc. I'm not sure why no one called the police. I'm just thankful I didn't hurt someone, including myself.

♥   What a strange few weeks for someone who is supposed to be in remission. I'm not sure that word holds meaning for those of us with an incurable disease. First, my ears started itching, followed by most of my skin. I have visible scratch marks on both of my thighs, from itching during the night. Adding to the misery, I have had nausea every day for the past several weeks. All the while, my liver counts were escalating and I've learned that the Hepatitis C I never knew I had - nor how I got it - needs to be treated, IF my insurance company will pay for the $1,000/day pill for a period of 12 weeks. ($84,000) But it's the fatigue that got me this week - and I passed out while driving my car and rear-ended the vehicle in front of me. I must have been in and out of consciousness for most of the ride home from the clinic because at the scene of the accident the driver of another vehicle screamed out his window at me - hey lady - that I should get off the road because before I finally hit someone, I had been swerving up onto curbs and nearly clipped a few trees. And I now understand the meaning of that gut feeling I've had that I need to get a second opinion and most likely a new oncologist. Anyway, my wings have been clipped - no more driving for now.

I have an appointment with my Palliative Care doctor this morning to hash over all these symptoms, and to ask for her advice on getting a new doctor. PS - my best advice if you ever see a vehicle driving erratically, call the police. I feel sick to know how far I might have been driving without the mental capacity to safely do so. We always assume it might be someone on their cell phone or a drunk. That's not always the case - it could be someone, like me, having a health crisis. Hope everyone is in good shape today. Big hugs all around.

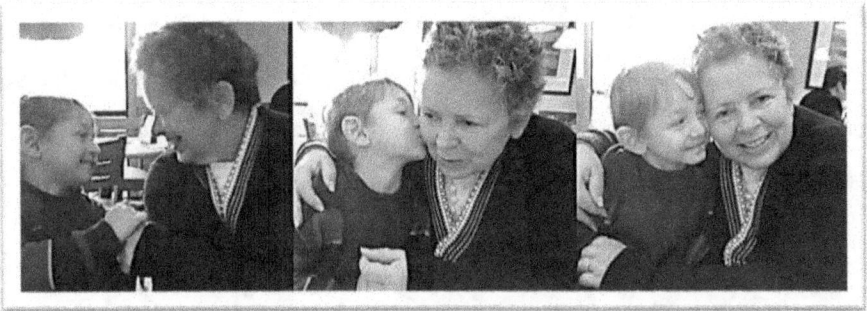

♥   News to report - there were 9 white blood cells in my spinal fluid so they will start me on an antibiotic while trying to figure out whether the infection is in my brain or elsewhere. It may or may not be good news - but I am glad to know there is a reason for what has been happening.

♥   I finally had my first out-patient infusion of Rituxan, first of two years' worth. Three and 1/2 hours closer to ... what? Oh, ya - fighting for my life without knowing how long I have or how good it's going to be. And yet, I go through the motions with the best of intentions because living is all I know how to do. Dying is not an option. I mean, what if I screw up - it's not like I get a second or third chance. But - living - now that's what I know. So, cheers, my friends -- here's to living! (P.S. I'm toasting with a 5-oz. box of Milk Duds, and just the slightest hint of perverted humor.)

♥ One of the things I used to do was rearrange my furniture a lot. Made everyone think I was a bit cuckoo, but it gave me a feeling of satisfaction - that I had control of something. Of course, I've been too weak or tired to do this for the past 11 months -- but yesterday, I suddenly had a hankering to be in control of something. And I moved furniture... for 2 1/2 hours... cleaning while I moved stuff. My little old 1940's house has an ambiguous floor plan - is it the living or dining room, and vice versa? Switched ALL the furniture, by myself, from one room to the other. While I was so sore and exhausted by the time I finished -- it felt GREAT to be able to do it, by myself. And I am once again in control.

♥ I fell asleep last night eating a bologna sandwich. The bologna is long gone - thanks to my two canine vultures, but the bread with mustard remain... well, much of the mustard turned up on my face. Hope everyone had a good night's rest, or that our friends who are just entering nighttime had a great day. Hugs.

♥ My friend Phil just completed his 12th round of Hyper-CVAD. He's relapsed twice. We both have Blastoid, and were diagnosed a few weeks apart. I've known him for 30 years. Irony. I know that 12 rounds of chemo can't be good for one's body. Phil — I want you to know that we're still in this together. Hold on.

♥ Isn't it interesting that we get so consumed with treatment that we sometimes forget to enjoy the moment we're in? I mean, when I was told I had to stop chemo because I wasn't recovering well enough in between, I was like, OK, but now what do I do? I went from being in the hospital on a regular basis, going in for labs 3 times a week, to practically nothing. So, then I was finally able to begin Rituxan. The plan, every other month. Labs, monthly. I went from nearly a year of intense medical care to feeling like a fraud! I think this is the point where we think, okay well I should have SCT or something else. No, Linda Marie, this is where you change pace and just enjoy the fact that you're still alive, feeling not as badly as you felt before, and try to stop thinking of death. Easier said than done. But, time passes, and it gets easier to just live in the moment, and be thankful. I am alive... so are you.

I enjoy reading your posts, Linda. You make me laugh and cry. I look forward to reading your book. The funny things that happened to me during chemo were, one day I decided to cook in a Webber (first time effort). Now, I had no hair, but I was very proud of my make up efforts and I still felt pretty. Anyway, I lit the beads and put the lid on after it was lit. Silly me, I didn't open the vents, so it was starting to catch fire. In a panic, I took off the lid to save my handles from melting... and POOF! Eyebrows and eyelashes gone! Hahahahaha it was so funny that the chemo didn't have the chance to remove then. I did it myself! -Sharon

FINAL THOUGHTS

How can one possibly cope with the demands and pressures of being diagnosed with a deadly illness? The question more appropriately should be, how can one not? Each day at the forefront of my mind is the reality that this disease will kill me, even though the timeline is unknown. Yet, dwelling on the inevitable isn't going to help me live. So, how does one create a habit of positive living during such difficulties? Simple to me, one must prepare for dying so that living can be in the present mind.

Will there be bad days? Absolutely! And there are bits and pieces of those bad days immersed in every day. As I told my son, I can't not think about dying when it's in my head. But I'm also alive, making plans, thinking of ways to positively impact life in my circle of influence, knowing it will be my legacy.

Another important aspect of my life is to be aware of and tuned into those around me. So, who have I been surrounded by? Cancer patients, caregivers and medical staff, all of whom must find a balance in living with sickness. Some are far better than others. I consider them to be the ones who aren't afraid to confess that they're having a bad day, to own those feelings. And those bad days aren't superficial. They are deeply embedded in our minds, hearts and souls. Yet cancer patients also must have a sense of hope, or they wouldn't get out of bed each morning. We must create a path that is ours, and not be afraid of criticism.

I hate having cancer and knowing I will die. But this illness has been the ultimate blessing for me. It caused me to look up from what I once thought was important in time to learn that my priorities needed to change.

One hundred nine people visited me during my first months of chemotherapy. I didn't know that many people even liked me! Before, I was living under the radar. Now I am fully alive and aware of every emotion, every pain, sorrow, hurt, and love. Every nerve is sitting right under the skin, like receptors ready to absorb the energy around me. I am more alive – and unafraid – now than ever before.

It's this new way of living that creates potential in each day. I can see the beauty in each moment, the vibrant colors surrounding me... the sounds of nature. The love of a friend, and the touch of a hug – all are bigger than ever, and invoke memories I've long since forgotten.

It's important to me that people I love understand and accept the reality that I am going to die from my cancer. I know their instinct is to offer a plethora of good intentions, but I need for my own emotional well-being for my friends and family to be grounded. I have the truth, and I want to live in it. Cancer is not a pretend sickness that if we all wish hard enough will go away. Maybe there will be an unexpected miracle that will save my life, but offering me that potential in every single conversation is not welcome. Finding something meaningful to do while living with an illness that causes you to change your lifestyle is so important. I have been on medical leave from a job which held great meaning for me, one that filled my need to help others, to stay busy, to be engaged in my community. So, I went in search of volunteer positions that wouldn't require a huge time commitment, yet would feed my soul.

Look for things you love to do. Don't spend your time just doing – but loving what you're doing. I've also written 3 poems, and my cousin has set them to music. I've shared them with the hospital's music therapy program, which in turn is sharing them with patients throughout the hospital. Finally, I always wanted to write a book. I don't know whether I'm any good at it, but I wrote this book to share with others who are going through life changing illness, such as cancer. By no means do I know all there is about anything relevant to cancer. But I do know that I'm a warrior, that I've managed to survive the day to day challenges I have faced through my personal journey with cancer. I hope somehow what I've expressed and experienced has resonated with you. Accept the challenge of living with cancer with as much grace as you can muster. For some it will be a long journey, but regardless of your diagnosis or prognosis, make it the journey of a lifetime. You are surrounded by knowledgeable medical professionals, and the love of family and friends. Rest when you need to; ask for what you need; and, scream when it becomes necessary. You are the director, you make the decisions that feel right for you, and you can decide how the rest of your life will be. Make it a life well-lived, one day at a time.

Oh, my friend, it's not what they take away from you that counts — it's what you do with what you have left.

Hubert Humphrey

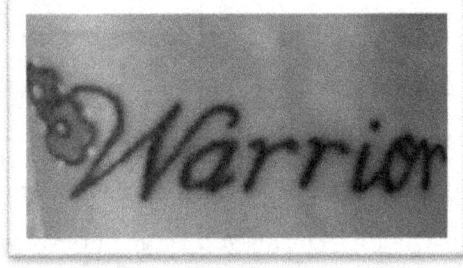

I went to Las Vegas for a couple of days with friends, and came home with my first tattoo. It is very symbolic to me. Think outside the box, my friends. Don't be afraid to be in the moment, to express yourself in meaningful ways. Be brave. You are a warrior!   - LT

Epilogue

On October 30, 2016 at 2:08 AM, my cancer buddy and long-time friend, Phil Johnson passed away. Phil and I met many years ago when he was the mailman who delivered to an office building I managed. He was such a likeable guy that one couldn't help but gravitate towards him. Then when our kids started school, his son Evan and my son John joined T-Ball, and Phil was their coach.

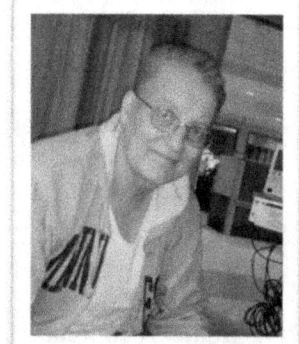

When I was admitted into the hospital to begin my chemotherapy, I found Phil again. It was rather silly. I was wandering like a deer in headlights when I heard from behind me, "Mailman coming."

Phil and I were diagnosed a month apart with the same aggressive cancer that I've written about in these pages. We were both patients of the Frauenshuh Cancer Center in St. Louis Park, MN; we both admitted to Methodist Hospital for in-patient treatment, and both had the same oncologist. Too much coincidence.

Phil showed me the ropes during my first hospital stay. He was so strong and easy-going, and I learned a lot from him. We were likely the oncology nurses' worse nightmare, as we were always together and loved to tag-team. I think we all became like family over the months of hospitalizations, and it was just a given that Phil would be having his coffee in my room first thing in the morning, and we would wander the halls out of boredom.

When Phil relapsed for the second time, I stopped crying and became protective. We talked with doctors together, asked questions together. We were fighting to stay alive and maintain a quality of life.

Live every single day to its fullest. Love like there is no tomorrow, and never miss an opportunity to walk in the sunshine, listen to the sound of the wind in the autumn leaves, or hold the hand of a friend. Today is all any of us may have. I was lucky to travel through most of my journey with a friend like Phil. He filled my heart with glitter and gold.

ARA-C: Cytarabine or cytosine arabinoside (Cytosar-U or Depocyt) is a chemotherapy agent used mainly in the treatment of cancers of white blood cells such as acute myeloid leukemia (AML) and non-Hodgkin lymphoma. It is also known as *ara-C* (arabinofuranosyl cytidine).

American Cancer Society: Dedicated to helping persons who face *cancer*. Supports research, patient services, early detection, treatment and education. Cancer.org

Ativan: a benzodiazepine used to treat anxiety.

Bone Marrow Biopsy: A bone marrow biopsy is part of a bone marrow test that takes a sample of your solid bone tissue. This test looks for abnormalities in your blood cells and signs of any diseases.

CT Scan: A computerized tomography (CT) scan combines a series of X-ray images taken from different angles and uses computer processing to create cross-sectional images, or slices, of the bones, blood vessels and soft tissues inside your body. CT scan images provide more detailed information than plain X-rays do.

Cancer Rehab: Physical *rehabilitation* to help your body recover from *cancer*

Doxorubicin: *Doxorubicin*, sold under the trade names Adriamycin among others, is a medication used in cancer chemotherapy.

Dilaudid: *Dilaudid* (hydromorphone) is an opioid pain medication.

GI: Gastroenterologists have extensive training in the diagnosis and treatment of conditions that affect the esophagus, stomach, small intestine, large intestine (colon), and biliary system (e.g., liver, pancreas, gallbladder, bile ducts). Gastroenterology is a subspecialty of internal medicine.

Hypoactive Delirium: Patients with hyperactive delirium demonstrate features of restlessness, agitation and hyper vigilance and often experience hallucinations and delusions. By contrast, patients with hypoactive delirium present with lethargy and sedation, respond slowly to questioning, and show little spontaneous movement.

Health Care Directive: A *health care directive* is a written document that informs other of your wishes about your *health care*. It allows you to name a person ("agent") to decide for you if you are unable to decide. It also allows you to name an agent if you want someone else to decide for you.

Hepatitis C: An infection caused by a virus that attacks the liver and leads to inflammation.

HyperCVAD: The term 'hyper' refers to the hyperfractionated nature of the chemotherapy, which is given in smaller doses, more frequently, to minimize side effects. 'CVAD' is the acronym of the drugs used in course A: cyclophosphamide, vincristine, doxorubicin (also known by its trade name, Adriamycin), and dexamethasone.

Hickman: A Hickman line is a central venous catheter most often used for the administration of chemotherapy or other medications, as well as for the withdrawal of blood for analysis.

Leukemia and Lymphoma Society: LLS exists to find cures and ensure access to treatments for blood cancer patients. We are the voice for all blood cancer patients and we work to ensure access to treatments for all blood cancer patients. Lls.org

Lumbar Puncture: the procedure of taking fluid from the spine in the lower back through a hollow needle, usually done for diagnostic purposes.

MRI: Magnetic resonance imaging (*MRI*) is a noninvasive medical test that physicians use to diagnose and treat medical conditions. *MRI* uses a powerful magnetic field, radio frequency pulses and a computer to produce detailed pictures of organs, soft tissues, bone and virtually all other internal body structures.

MTX: Methotrexate; chemotherapy and immunosuppressant

PET Scan: A positron emission tomography (PET) scan is an imaging test that allows your doctor to check for diseases in your body. The scan uses a special dye that has radioactive tracers. These tracers are injected into a vein in your arm. Your organs and tissues then absorb the tracer.

Platelets: a small colorless disk-shaped cell fragment without a nucleus, found in large numbers in blood and involved in clotting.

Palliative Care: Palliative care (pronounced pal-lee-uh-tiv) is specialized medical care for people with serious illness. It focuses on providing relief from the symptoms and stress of a serious illness. The goal is to improve quality of life for both the patient and the family.

POLST: *Physicians Orders for Life Sustaining Treatment (POLST)* is a legal document stating the type of care a person would like in an emergency medical situation. It should be posted so paramedics can easily find it when responding to a medical emergency at your home.

Rituxan: Rituximab is a monoclonal antibody against the protein CD20, which is primarily found on the surface of immune system B cells.

Richter's Transformation: *Richter's* Syndrome (RS), is a rare complication of Chronic Lymphocytic Leukaemia (CLL) and/or Small Lymphocytic Lymphoma (SLL) characterised by the sudden *transformation* of the CLL/SLL into a significantly more aggressive form of large cell lymphoma. *Chronic lymphocytic leukemia (CLL)* is a type of cancer that starts from cells that become certain white blood cells (called lymphocytes) in the bone marrow. The cancer (leukemia) cells start in the bone marrow but then go into the blood. *Diffuse large B-cell lymphoma (DLBCL or DLBL)* is a cancer of B cells, a type of white blood cell responsible for producing antibodies.

Stem Cell Transplant: A bone marrow transplant is a procedure that infuses healthy blood stem cells into your body to replace your damaged or diseased bone marrow. A bone marrow transplant is also called a stem cell transplant.

WBC: *White blood cells* (WBCs) are an important part of the immune system. They help fight infections by attacking bacteria, viruses, and germs that invade the body.

There is financial support available to those in need. How much and where it comes from can be a challenge to explore. Please plan to meet with Palliative Care at your health care facility. Palliative care (pronounced pal-lee-uh-tiv) is specialized medical care for people with serious illness. It focuses on providing relief from the symptoms and stress of a serious illness. The goal is to improve quality of life for both the patient and the family. The social workers can help with POLST, Health Care Directives, and more, and they all follow your care once you become a Palliative Care patient.

Special thanks

to those who have helped me function throughout my journey, giving me rides, bringing meals, taking me shopping or to dinner, having long conversations about life and death and all that comes in between. While I have so many people to be thankful for, I want to call out a special few:

John Trummer	Janet Prchal
Ken & Bridget Gothberg	Deb Sparling & Jeff Jacobs
Anna Alberto	Mark Schwartz
Mark Nevermann	Mike Spencer
Josh & Susan Schneck	Randy Trummer

St. Louis Park Sunrise Rotary Club

Frauenshuh Cancer Center & Methodist Hospital

A PLACE FOR YOUR SPECIAL THOUGHTS

_____

_____

_____

_____

_____

_____

_____

_____

_____

_____

_____

_____

_____

_____

_____

_____

_____

_____

_____

_____

_____

_____

_____

_____

_____

_____

www.ingramcontent.com/pod-product-compliance
Lightning Source LLC
Chambersburg PA
CBHW070232290526
45789CB00004B/1596